The Essential Guide to Managing Diabetes

A Comprehensive Handbook for Optimal Health and Wellness

Brian Abby

Table of Contents

Brian Abby

Table of Contents

Brian Abby

Introduction

Welcome to "The Essential Guide to Managing Diabetes: A Comprehensive Handbook for Optimal Health and Wellness." This book is your go-to resource for understanding and effectively managing diabetes to live a healthy and fulfilling life.

The Importance of Managing Diabetes

Diabetes is a chronic condition that affects millions of people worldwide. When left unmanaged, it can lead to serious health complications, including heart disease, kidney problems, nerve damage, and vision impairment. However, with the right knowledge, tools, and strategies, you can take control of your diabetes and minimize the risk of complications.

Empowering Yourself with Knowledge

This comprehensive handbook is designed to empower you with the knowledge and skills needed to effectively manage your diabetes. Whether you have been recently diagnosed or have been living with diabetes for a while, this guide will provide you with practical information, evidence-based strategies, and valuable insights to support your journey towards optimal health and wellness.

A Holistic Approach to Diabetes Management

Managing diabetes goes beyond simply monitoring blood sugar levels. It involves adopting a holistic approach that encompasses various aspects of your lifestyle, including nutrition, physical activity, medication management, stress reduction, and self-care practices. This handbook will guide you through each of these areas, offering practical tips and advice to help you make informed decisions and take proactive steps towards better health.

Understanding Diabetes Types and Treatment Options

Diabetes is not a one-size-fits-all condition. There are different types of diabetes, including type 1, type 2, gestational diabetes, and other less common types. Understanding the characteristics and treatment options for each type is crucial for effective management. This guide will provide you with an in-depth understanding of the various diabetes types, their causes, symptoms, and recommended treatment approaches.

Your Journey to Optimal Health and Wellness

Managing diabetes can sometimes feel overwhelming, but with the right information and support, you can navigate this journey successfully. This guide will be your trusted companion, offering practical strategies, lifestyle recommendations, and expert advice to help you achieve optimal health and wellness.

Throughout the following chapters, we will delve into topics such as understanding diabetes, nutrition and diet, physical activity, medication management, blood sugar monitoring, managing diabetes in everyday life, preventive care, support resources, and more. Each chapter will provide valuable insights and actionable steps to help you navigate the complexities of diabetes management with confidence.

Remember, managing diabetes is a lifelong commitment, but it doesn't mean you can't live a fulfilling life. By taking control of your health and implementing the strategies outlined in this guide, you can thrive while effectively managing your diabetes.

Let's embark on this journey together and discover the essential knowledge and tools you need for optimal health and wellness with diabetes management.

Chapter 1: Understanding Diabetes

In this chapter, we will explore the fundamentals of diabetes, including its definition, types, causes, symptoms, and methods of diagnosis. Understanding the intricacies of diabetes is essential for effectively managing the condition and making informed decisions about your health.

Definition of Diabetes

Diabetes is a chronic metabolic disorder characterized by high blood sugar levels (hyperglycemia). It occurs when the body either doesn't produce enough insulin or is unable to effectively utilize the insulin it produces. Insulin, a hormone produced by the pancreas, regulates the absorption of glucose into the cells to provide them with energy.

Types of Diabetes

There are three main types of diabetes:

1. Type 1 Diabetes: Also known as insulin-dependent diabetes, type 1 diabetes is an autoimmune condition in which the body's immune system mistakenly attacks and destroys the insulin-producing cells in the pancreas. People with type 1 diabetes require lifelong insulin therapy.

2. Type 2 Diabetes: Type 2 diabetes is the most common kind of diabetes, accounting for the majority of cases. It occurs when the body becomes resistant to insulin or doesn't produce enough insulin to meet its needs. Type

2 diabetes is often associated with lifestyle factors such as obesity, sedentary behavior, and poor dietary choices.

3. Gestational Diabetes: Gestational diabetes develops during pregnancy and usually resolves after childbirth. It affects women who did not have diabetes before pregnancy. However, women with gestational diabetes have an increased risk of developing type 2 diabetes later in life.

Causes and Risk Factors

The causes of diabetes vary depending on the type:

- Type 1 Diabetes: The exact cause of type 1 diabetes is unknown, but it is believed to involve a combination of genetic and environmental factors.

- Type 2 Diabetes: Type 2 diabetes is influenced by multiple factors, including genetics, lifestyle choices, and underlying medical conditions such as obesity and insulin resistance.

- Gestational Diabetes: Hormonal changes during pregnancy can interfere with insulin function, leading to gestational diabetes. Risk factors for gestational diabetes include being overweight, having a family history of diabetes, and advanced maternal age.

Common Symptoms

While the symptoms may differ among the types of diabetes, there are common signs to be aware of:

- Frequent urination

- Excessive thirst

- Unexplained weight loss

- Fatigue

- Increased hunger

- Blurred vision

- Slow-healing wounds

- Recurring infections, particularly in the urinary tract or skin

If you experience any of these symptoms, it is essential to consult your healthcare provider for a proper diagnosis.

Diagnosis of Diabetes

Diagnosing diabetes involves various tests to measure blood sugar levels:

- Fasting Plasma Glucose (FPG) Test: This test measures blood sugar levels after an overnight fast. A fasting plasma glucose level of 126 milligrams per deciliter (mg/dL) or higher on two separate occasions is indicative of diabetes.

- Oral Glucose Tolerance Test (OGTT): The OGTT involves measuring blood sugar levels before and two hours after consuming a glucose-rich drink. A two-hour blood glucose level of 200 mg/dL or higher indicates diabetes.

- Hemoglobin A1C (HbA1c) Test: The HbA1c test provides an average blood sugar level over the past two to three months. An HbA1c level of 6.5% or higher is indicative of diabetes.

Proper diagnosis is crucial to determine the appropriate treatment plan for managing diabetes effectively.

In the next chapter, we will delve deeper into the impact of diabetes on health and the importance of proactive management to prevent complications and achieve optimal well-being.

Chapter 2: The Impact of Diabetes on Health

In this chapter, we will explore the wide-ranging impact that diabetes can have on your overall health and well-being. Understanding these potential complications will underscore the importance of effectively managing diabetes to prevent long-term health problems.

Complications Associated with Diabetes

When diabetes is left unmanaged or poorly controlled, it can lead to various complications that affect different parts of the body. Some common complications include:

1. Cardiovascular Disease: Diabetes increases the risk of heart disease,

heart attack, stroke, and other cardiovascular conditions. Elevated blood sugar levels, high blood pressure, and abnormal cholesterol levels contribute to the increased risk.

2. Kidney Disease: Diabetes can damage the kidneys over time, leading to diabetic nephropathy. If left untreated, it can progress to chronic kidney disease and kidney failure, requiring dialysis or a kidney transplant.

3. Nerve Damage (Neuropathy): Elevated blood sugar levels can cause damage to the nerves, leading to symptoms such as numbness, tingling, pain, and loss of sensation in the extremities. Neuropathy can also

affect other organs, such as the digestive system and the urinary tract.

4. Eye Complications: Diabetes increases the risk of eye conditions such as diabetic retinopathy, cataracts, and glaucoma. Diabetic retinopathy, characterized by damage to the blood vessels in the retina, is a leading cause of vision loss and blindness among people with diabetes.

5. Foot Problems: Diabetes can impair blood circulation and nerve function in the feet, leading to foot ulcers, infections, and, in severe cases, amputations. Proper foot care and regular examinations are crucial for preventing complications.

6. Skin Conditions: People with diabetes are more prone to skin conditions, including bacterial and fungal infections, as well as dry, itchy skin. High blood sugar levels and impaired immune function contribute to these skin-related issues.

7. Mental Health Challenges: Diabetes management can impact mental well-being, leading to stress, anxiety, depression, and diabetes-related distress. It is important to address these psychological aspects and seek support when needed.

Importance of Diabetes Management

By effectively managing diabetes, you can significantly reduce the risk of complications and improve your overall health and well-being. Proper management strategies may include:

- Blood Sugar Control: Keeping your blood sugar levels within the target range recommended by your healthcare provider is crucial for preventing complications.

- Healthy Eating: Adopting a balanced and nutritious diet that focuses on whole foods, portion control, and appropriate carbohydrate intake can help manage blood sugar levels and support overall health.

- Regular Physical Activity: Engaging in regular exercise and physical activity helps improve insulin sensitivity, maintain a healthy weight, and promote cardiovascular health.

- Medication Management: Taking prescribed medications, such as insulin or oral hypoglycemic agents, as directed by your healthcare provider, is essential for controlling blood sugar levels.

- Routine Monitoring: Regularly monitoring blood sugar levels, blood pressure, cholesterol levels, and other relevant markers enables you to track your progress and make necessary adjustments to your treatment plan.

- Healthcare Team Collaboration: Working closely with your healthcare team, including doctors, diabetes educators, and specialists, ensures comprehensive care and guidance tailored to your specific needs.

Taking Control of Your Diabetes

Managing diabetes requires a proactive approach and ongoing commitment. By taking control of your diabetes management, you can minimize the risk of complications, optimize your health, and lead a fulfilling life.

In the next chapter, we will discuss the goals of diabetes management and how to set realistic targets for achieving optimal health and wellness.

Chapter 3: Setting Goals for Diabetes Management

In this chapter, we will discuss the importance of setting goals for diabetes management and explore key areas where goals can make a positive impact on your health and well-being.

1. Blood Sugar Level Targets

Maintaining target blood sugar levels is crucial for effective diabetes management. Setting specific goals for blood sugar control can help you monitor and regulate your condition more effectively. Consider the following blood sugar level targets:

- Fasting Blood Glucose: Set a goal to maintain your fasting blood glucose level within a specific range, such as 80-130 mg/dL (4.4-7.2 mmol/L).

- Postprandial Blood Glucose: Aim to keep your blood sugar levels within the target range 1-2 hours after meals, typically below 180 mg/dL (10 mmol/L).

- HbA1c: HbA1c is a measure of your average blood glucose levels over the past three months. Set a target HbA1c level, such as below 7% or as advised by your healthcare provider.

Monitoring your blood sugar levels regularly and working towards achieving these targets can help you better manage your diabetes and reduce the risk of complications.

2. Preventing and Managing Complications

Another essential aspect of diabetes management is preventing and managing potential complications. Establishing goals in this area can help you take proactive steps to safeguard your health. Consider the following goals:

- Eye Health: Schedule regular eye examinations to monitor for diabetic retinopathy and other diabetes-related eye conditions. Aim to have a comprehensive eye exam at least once a year.

- Kidney Health: Focus on maintaining healthy kidney function by controlling blood pressure and blood sugar levels. Set a goal to undergo regular urine and blood tests to monitor kidney health.

- Foot Care: Establish a goal to conduct daily foot inspections, keep your feet clean and moisturized, and wear comfortable, well-fitting shoes to prevent foot ulcers and infections.

- Heart Health: Adopt heart-healthy habits, such as maintaining a healthy weight, eating a balanced diet, engaging in regular physical activity, managing blood pressure and cholesterol levels, and quitting smoking if applicable.

Working towards these goals can significantly reduce the risk of complications associated with diabetes and promote overall well-being.

3. Adopting a Healthy Lifestyle

Embracing a healthy lifestyle is key to managing diabetes effectively. By setting goals related to your lifestyle choices, you can make positive changes that support your overall health. Consider the following goals:

- Healthy Eating: Set a goal to follow a balanced diet rich in fruits, vegetables, whole grains, lean proteins, and healthy fats. Limit the intake of processed foods, sugary snacks, and beverages.

- Physical Activity: Establish a goal to engage in regular physical activity, such as walking, jogging, swimming, or cycling. Aim for at least 150 minutes of moderate-intensity exercise each week.

- Weight Management: If necessary, set a realistic weight loss or weight maintenance goal. Consult with a healthcare professional or registered dietitian to develop a personalized plan.

- Stress Management: Adopt stress management techniques such as deep breathing exercises, meditation, yoga, or engaging in hobbies and activities that promote relaxation.

By setting and working towards these lifestyle goals, you can improve your overall health, better manage your diabetes, and enhance your quality of life.

Chapter 4: Nutrition and Diabetes

In this chapter, we will explore the crucial role of nutrition in managing diabetes effectively. Making informed and healthy food choices can help control blood sugar levels, maintain a healthy weight, and prevent complications associated with diabetes.

Understanding Carbohydrates, Proteins, and Fats

To effectively manage diabetes, it's important to understand the role of different macronutrients:

1. Carbohydrates: Carbohydrates have the most significant impact on blood sugar levels. They are the body's primary source of energy. It's important for individuals with

diabetes to understand how different types of carbohydrates affect their blood sugar levels. Focus on consuming complex carbohydrates, such as whole grains, legumes, vegetables, and fruits, which provide fiber and essential nutrients.

2. Proteins: Proteins are essential for building and repairing tissues, supporting immune function, and providing a source of energy. Choose lean sources of protein, such as poultry, fish, tofu, legumes, and low-fat dairy products. These options are lower in saturated fats and can help manage weight and control blood sugar levels.

3. Fats: Healthy fats play a crucial role in the body, providing energy, supporting cell growth, and aiding in the absorption of fat-soluble vitamins. Choose sources of unsaturated fats, such as avocados, nuts, seeds, and olive oil. Limit saturated and trans fats, found in fatty meats, full-fat dairy products, and processed foods, as they can increase the risk of heart disease.

Meal Planning and Portion Control

Meal planning and portion control are essential for managing diabetes. Here are some strategies to consider:

1. Create a Meal Plan: Develop a structured meal plan that includes a balance of carbohydrates, proteins, and fats. Consider working with a

registered dietitian or diabetes educator to tailor a meal plan to your specific needs and preferences.

2. Carbohydrate Counting: Carbohydrate counting is a method that involves estimating the number of carbohydrates in each meal and adjusting insulin or medication doses accordingly. Learn how to count carbohydrates and work with your healthcare team to determine the appropriate carbohydrate intake for your individual needs.

3. Portion Control: Be mindful of portion sizes to avoid overeating. Use measuring cups, food scales, or visual cues to ensure you're consuming appropriate portions. Consider using

smaller plates and bowls to help control portion sizes visually.

4. Regular Meal Patterns: Establish regular meal patterns and aim to eat at consistent times throughout the day. Spacing out meals evenly can help regulate blood sugar levels and prevent extreme fluctuations.

Healthy Eating Strategies

In addition to understanding macronutrients and practicing portion control, incorporating healthy eating strategies can further enhance diabetes management:

1. Fiber-Rich Foods: Include plenty of fiber-rich foods in your diet, such as whole grains, legumes, fruits, and vegetables. Fiber helps regulate blood

sugar levels, promotes satiety, and supports digestive health.

2. Hydration: Stay hydrated by drinking plenty of water throughout the day. Water helps maintain overall health and can assist in managing blood sugar levels. Limit sugary beverages and alcohol, as they can lead to blood sugar spikes and affect hydration.

3. Meal Timing and Snacking: Consider spacing out meals and snacks to maintain consistent blood sugar levels. Aim for a balance of carbohydrates, proteins, and fats in each meal and snack to provide sustained energy and prevent blood sugar fluctuations.

4. Mindful Eating: Practice mindful eating by savoring each bite, eating slowly, and paying attention to hunger and fullness cues. This can help prevent overeating and promote a healthier relationship with food.

By incorporating these strategies into your daily routine, you can create a balanced and nutritious diet that supports optimal diabetes management.

Proper nutrition plays a vital role in managing diabetes effectively. Understanding carbohydrates, proteins, and fats, implementing portion control, and adopting healthy eating strategies can help control blood sugar levels, maintain a healthy weight, and reduce the risk of complications associated with diabetes.

In the next chapter, we will explore the importance of physical activity and its significant benefits in diabetes management.

Chapter 5: Physical Activity and Exercise

Physical activity and exercise are essential components of managing diabetes effectively. Engaging in regular exercise offers numerous benefits, including improved blood sugar control, weight management, increased energy levels, enhanced cardiovascular health, and reduced risk of complications. In this chapter, we will explore the benefits of exercise for diabetes management, provide guidance on creating an exercise plan, and discuss strategies for incorporating physical activity into your daily life.

Benefits of Exercise for Diabetes Management

1. Improved Blood Sugar Control: Exercise helps lower blood sugar levels by increasing insulin sensitivity and allowing glucose to be used for energy. It can also reduce insulin resistance, which is beneficial for individuals with type 2 diabetes. Regular exercise helps stabilize blood sugar levels and can lead to better overall diabetes management.

2. Weight Management: Physical activity and exercise play a crucial role in weight management. By burning calories and promoting fat loss, exercise can help achieve and maintain a healthy weight.

Maintaining a healthy weight is important for diabetes management, as excess weight can contribute to insulin resistance and difficulties in blood sugar control.

3. Cardiovascular Health: Regular exercise strengthens the heart and improves cardiovascular health. It helps lower blood pressure, reduce bad cholesterol (LDL) levels, and increase good cholesterol (HDL) levels. These benefits are particularly important for individuals with diabetes, as they have a higher risk of developing heart disease.

4. Increased Energy Levels: Engaging in physical activity boosts energy levels and reduces feelings of fatigue.

Exercise improves circulation, increases oxygen delivery to the body's tissues, and enhances overall stamina. Regular exercise can help individuals with diabetes combat the tiredness often associated with the condition.

5. Stress Reduction: Exercise is a great stress reliever. Physical activity stimulates the production of endorphins, which are natural mood boosters. Regular exercise can reduce stress, anxiety, and depression, promoting mental well-being and overall quality of life.

Creating an Exercise Plan

Developing an exercise plan tailored to your needs and preferences is essential for long-term success. Here are some steps to consider when creating an exercise plan:

1. Consult Your Healthcare Provider: Before starting an exercise program, consult your healthcare provider. They can provide guidance based on your individual health status and any specific considerations related to diabetes management.

2. Set Realistic Goals: Set achievable goals that align with your fitness level and lifestyle. Consider factors such as the type of exercise, duration, frequency, and intensity. Gradually increase the intensity and duration of your workouts over time.

3. Choose Activities You Enjoy: Select activities that you find enjoyable and

that fit your interests and abilities. This will increase your motivation and likelihood of sticking with the exercise plan. Options can include walking, swimming, cycling, dancing, yoga, or group fitness classes.

4. Mix Cardiovascular and Strength Training: Include both cardiovascular exercises and strength training in your exercise plan. Cardiovascular exercises, such as brisk walking, jogging, or cycling, improve cardiovascular health and help with weight management. Strength training exercises, such as weightlifting or bodyweight exercises, help build muscle and increase metabolism.

5. Consider Flexibility and Balance: Incorporate flexibility exercises, such as stretching or yoga, to improve joint mobility and flexibility. Additionally, include balance exercises, such as tai chi or yoga, to improve stability and reduce the risk of falls.

6. Start Slowly and Progress Gradually: If you are new to exercise or have been inactive for a while, start with low-impact activities and gradually increase the intensity and duration. This approach allows your body to adapt and reduces the risk of injuries.

7. Monitor Your Blood Sugar: Pay attention to your blood sugar levels before, during, and after exercise. It's important to monitor how exercise

affects your blood sugar levels, especially if you take insulin or certain diabetes medications that can cause hypoglycemia (low blood sugar).

Incorporating Physical Activity into Daily Life

In addition to structured exercise sessions, finding ways to incorporate physical activity into your daily life can help you maintain an active lifestyle. Here are some strategies:

1. Take Frequent Walks: Walk whenever possible, whether it's taking a stroll during your lunch break, parking farther away from your destination, or opting for the stairs instead of the elevator. Walking is a low-impact activity that can be easily incorporated into your daily routine.

2. Make Active Social Plans: Plan social activities that involve physical activity. Instead of meeting friends for coffee, consider going for a hike, playing a sport together, or taking a dance class. This allows you to enjoy time with loved ones while also being active.

3. Use Active Transportation: Whenever feasible, choose active modes of transportation, such as walking or cycling, for short distances. This not only helps you stay active but also reduces your carbon footprint and contributes to environmental sustainability.

4. Take Active Breaks: If you have a sedentary job, take regular breaks to stretch, walk around, or perform

simple exercises. Set a reminder to get up and move every hour, even if it's just for a few minutes.

5. Join Fitness or Exercise Groups: Consider joining fitness or exercise groups in your community or online. This provides a supportive environment and opportunities to engage in group activities and classes.

Remember, consistency is key when it comes to physical activity and exercise. Aim for at least 150 minutes of moderate-intensity aerobic activity per week, spread out over several days, along with strength training exercises at least twice a week. Make it a priority to stay active and choose activities that you enjoy, ensuring long-term adherence to your exercise plan.

Chapter 6: Medications and Insulin Therapy

Medications and insulin therapy are vital components of diabetes management for many individuals. In this chapter, we will provide an overview of diabetes medications, discuss the different types of insulin and administration methods, and explore medication management and adherence strategies.

Overview of Diabetes Medications

There are various types of medications available to help manage diabetes. The choice of medication depends on the type of diabetes, individual health factors, and treatment goals. Here are some commonly used diabetes medications:

1. Metformin: Metformin is usually the first-line medication for type 2 diabetes. It helps lower blood sugar levels by reducing glucose production in the liver and increasing insulin sensitivity. Metformin is typically taken orally and is well-tolerated by most individuals.

2. Sulfonylureas: Sulfonylureas stimulate the pancreas to produce more insulin. These medications can be taken orally and are often prescribed for individuals with type 2 diabetes who cannot adequately control their blood sugar levels with lifestyle modifications alone.

3. DPP-4 Inhibitors: Dipeptidyl peptidase-4 (DPP-4) inhibitors help

lower blood sugar levels by blocking the enzyme responsible for breaking down incretin hormones. These hormones stimulate insulin release and reduce glucagon secretion. DPP-4 inhibitors are taken orally and are commonly used as an add-on therapy to other diabetes medications.

4. GLP-1 Receptor Agonists: Glucagon-like peptide-1 (GLP-1) receptor agonists mimic the action of incretin hormones. They stimulate insulin secretion, suppress glucagon release, slow gastric emptying, and promote satiety. GLP-1 receptor agonists are available as injectable medications and are often prescribed for individuals with type 2 diabetes

who require additional blood sugar control.

5. Insulin: Insulin is a hormone that regulates blood sugar levels. It is a crucial medication for individuals with type 1 diabetes, and it may also be prescribed for those with type 2 diabetes who cannot achieve adequate blood sugar control with oral medications. Insulin can be administered through injections using syringes, insulin pens, or insulin pumps.

Types of Insulin and Administration Methods

There are different types of insulin available, categorized based on their onset, peak, and duration of action. The common types of insulin include:

1. Rapid-Acting Insulin: Rapid-acting insulin begins to work within 15 minutes after injection and peaks within 1 to 2 hours. It has a duration of action of approximately 3 to 4 hours. This type of insulin is often used to cover mealtime blood sugar spikes.

2. Short-Acting Insulin: Short-acting insulin starts working within 30 minutes after injection, peaks within 2 to 3 hours, and has a duration of action of around 5 to 8 hours. It is commonly used before meals to control blood sugar levels.

3. Intermediate-Acting Insulin: Intermediate-acting insulin takes effect within 2 to 4 hours, peaks within 4 to 12 hours, and typically lasts for approximately 12 to 18 hours. This type of insulin is often combined with rapid-acting or short-acting insulin to provide basal (background) insulin coverage throughout the day.

4. Long-Acting Insulin: Long-acting insulin starts working several hours after injection and has a relatively flat and consistent effect for approximately 24 hours. It provides basal insulin coverage and helps maintain stable blood sugar levels between meals and overnight.

Insulin can be administered using various methods:

1. Syringes: Insulin can be drawn into syringes and injected subcutaneously (under the skin) at various injection sites, such as the abdomen, thighs, or buttocks.

2. Insulin Pens: Insulin pens are pre-filled devices that allow for accurate dosing. They use disposable needles and are convenient for self-administration.

3. Insulin Pumps: Insulin pumps are small devices that deliver a continuous infusion of insulin throughout the day. The pump is worn externally and connected to the body through a small tube and cannula. It provides precise

insulin delivery and allows for flexibility in insulin dosing.

4. Inhaled Insulin: Inhaled insulin is a newer form of insulin administration that involves inhaling powdered insulin through a device called an inhaler. It is an alternative option for individuals who have difficulty with injections.

Medication Management and Adherence

Proper medication management and adherence are crucial for effective diabetes management. Here are some strategies to help you manage your medications effectively:

1. Follow Healthcare Provider's Instructions: It is essential to follow your healthcare provider's instructions

regarding medication dosage, timing, and administration. Ask questions and seek clarification if you have any doubts or concerns.

2. Keep a Medication Schedule: Create a medication schedule or use a medication reminder app to help you stay organized and remember to take your medications on time. Set alarms or use pill organizers to ensure you don't miss any doses.

3. Learn About Potential Side Effects: Familiarize yourself with the potential side effects of your medications. If you experience any adverse effects, notify your healthcare provider promptly.

4. Maintain an Updated Medication List: Keep an updated list of all your

medications, including dosages and frequencies. This information will be helpful when consulting with healthcare providers or in case of emergencies.

5. Refill Medications in Advance: Make sure to refill your prescriptions before you run out of medication. Plan ahead to avoid any interruptions in your medication regimen.

6. Communicate with Your Healthcare Team: Stay in touch with your healthcare team and inform them about any changes in your health status or if you are experiencing difficulties with your medications. They can provide guidance and make

necessary adjustments to your treatment plan.

7. Engage in Self-Monitoring: Regularly monitor your blood sugar levels as advised by your healthcare provider. This helps you assess the effectiveness of your medications and make adjustments if needed.

Remember, medication management is a collaborative effort between you and your healthcare team. Open communication, adherence to prescribed treatment plans, and regular follow-up appointments are essential for optimal diabetes management.

Chapter 7: Monitoring Blood Sugar Levels

Monitoring blood sugar levels is a critical aspect of diabetes management. In this chapter, we will explore different glucose monitoring techniques, learn how to interpret blood sugar readings, and discuss the benefits of continuous glucose monitoring (CGM) systems.

Glucose Monitoring Techniques

There are several methods available for monitoring blood sugar levels. Here are some commonly used glucose monitoring techniques:

1. Fingerstick Blood Glucose Testing: Fingerstick blood glucose testing involves pricking the fingertip with a lancet to obtain a small blood sample.

The blood sample is then placed on a test strip and inserted into a glucose meter, which provides a blood sugar reading within seconds. This method is convenient, portable, and allows for immediate results.

2. Continuous Glucose Monitoring (CGM) Systems: CGM systems consist of a small sensor inserted under the skin, typically on the abdomen, that continuously measures glucose levels in the interstitial fluid. The sensor sends the data wirelessly to a receiver or smartphone, providing real-time glucose readings and trends. CGM systems offer the advantage of continuous monitoring without the need for frequent fingerstick tests.

3. Flash Glucose Monitoring: Flash glucose monitoring is similar to CGM systems but does not provide continuous real-time glucose readings. Instead, users scan the sensor with a reader device to obtain glucose readings and trends. Flash glucose monitoring offers convenience and eliminates the need for routine fingerstick testing.

4. Urine Glucose Testing: Urine glucose testing involves collecting a urine sample and using test strips to detect the presence of glucose. This method is less accurate than blood glucose testing and is not commonly recommended for routine monitoring. It may be used in specific situations

when blood glucose testing is not feasible.

Interpreting Blood Sugar Readings

Interpreting blood sugar readings is crucial for understanding your diabetes management and making necessary adjustments. Here are some general guidelines for interpreting blood sugar readings:

1. Fasting Blood Sugar (FBS): Fasting blood sugar refers to the blood sugar level measured after an overnight fast. In most cases, a target range of 80-130 mg/dL (4.4-7.2 mmol/L) is recommended for fasting blood sugar. However, individual targets may vary based on factors such as age, overall health, and diabetes treatment plan.

2. Postprandial Blood Sugar: Postprandial blood sugar refers to the blood sugar level measured after a meal. The target range for postprandial blood sugar levels is typically below 180 mg/dL (10 mmol/L) two hours after starting a meal. Again, individual targets may vary based on personal circumstances.

3. HbA1c: HbA1c is a blood test that provides an average blood sugar level over the past two to three months. It is expressed as a percentage. The American Diabetes Association recommends aiming for an HbA1c level below 7% for most individuals with diabetes. However, individual targets may vary based on factors such

as age, health status, and the presence of other medical conditions.

It's important to note that blood sugar targets and interpretation may vary based on individual circumstances and recommendations provided by healthcare professionals. Regular monitoring, tracking trends, and discussing your results with your healthcare team will help guide your diabetes management plan effectively.

Continuous Glucose Monitoring (CGM) Systems

Continuous glucose monitoring (CGM) systems offer a comprehensive view of blood sugar levels throughout the day and night. These systems provide real-time data, including glucose trends, rate of change, and alerts for high or low blood sugar levels. Here are some benefits of CGM systems:

1. Improved Diabetes Management: CGM systems provide valuable information on how food, physical activity, medication, and other factors impact blood sugar levels. This data enables individuals to make informed decisions about their diabetes management, leading to improved control and prevention of blood sugar fluctuations.

2. Hypoglycemia and Hyperglycemia Detection: CGM systems can detect patterns of hypoglycemia (low blood sugar) and hyperglycemia (high blood sugar). They provide alerts for both high and low blood sugar levels,

allowing for timely intervention and prevention of complications.

3. Insight into Overnight Blood Sugar Levels: CGM systems offer continuous monitoring during sleep, providing valuable information about overnight blood sugar levels and trends. This data helps identify nocturnal hypoglycemia or hyperglycemia episodes and guides treatment adjustments.

4. Reduced Fingerstick Testing: CGM systems significantly reduce the need for routine fingerstick blood glucose testing. While periodic calibration with fingerstick testing is still necessary, CGM systems offer a more

convenient and less invasive alternative for continuous monitoring.

It's important to work closely with your healthcare team to understand and interpret CGM data effectively. They can help you set appropriate blood sugar targets, customize alert settings, and provide guidance on diabetes management based on the CGM reports.

Chapter 8: Managing Diabetes in Everyday Life

Living with diabetes requires everyday management and adaptation. In this chapter, we will discuss coping strategies for stress and emotional challenges, provide tips for traveling with diabetes, and explore sick-day management techniques.

Coping with Stress and Emotional Challenges

Stress and emotional challenges can have a significant impact on diabetes management. Here are some strategies to help you cope with stress and maintain emotional well-being:

1. Recognize Stress Triggers: Identify the factors that trigger stress in your life, such as work pressure, relationship

issues, or financial concerns. Awareness of these triggers can help you develop effective coping mechanisms.

2. Practice Stress Management Techniques: Engage in stress management techniques like deep breathing exercises, meditation, yoga, or physical activity. These activities can help reduce stress levels and promote relaxation.

3. Seek Support: Share your feelings and concerns with trusted family members, friends, or a support group. Connecting with others who understand your experiences can provide emotional support and practical advice.

4. Prioritize Self-Care: Take care of yourself by prioritizing self-care activities. This includes getting enough sleep, eating a balanced diet, engaging in regular physical activity, and practicing hobbies or activities you enjoy.

5. Talk to a Mental Health Professional: If you are struggling with significant emotional challenges or finding it difficult to cope with stress, consider seeking professional help from a mental health counselor or therapist who specializes in diabetes care.

Remember, managing your emotional well-being is just as important as managing your blood sugar levels. Taking care of your mental health can positively impact your overall diabetes management.

Traveling with Diabetes

Traveling can be enjoyable, but it also requires careful planning and preparation, especially when you have diabetes. Here are some tips to help you navigate travel while effectively managing your diabetes:

1. Pack Extra Supplies: Pack more than enough diabetes supplies, including insulin, oral medications, glucose meters, test strips, and syringes or pen needles. Consider carrying a backup glucose meter and extra batteries as well.

2. Carry Prescriptions and Medical Information: Keep a list of your medications, including generic names,

dosages, and prescriptions. Additionally, carry a document that outlines your medical history, emergency contacts, and any relevant allergies or medical conditions.

3. Plan for Time Zone Changes: If you are traveling across different time zones, consult with your healthcare provider on how to adjust your medication and insulin schedules accordingly. Proper planning can help prevent disruptions in your diabetes management.

4. Stay Hydrated and Mindful of Food Choices: Drink plenty of water and stay hydrated throughout your journey. Be mindful of your food choices, especially if you have specific

dietary requirements. Opt for balanced meals and snacks to maintain stable blood sugar levels.

5. Carry Snacks for Hypoglycemia: Pack some snacks like glucose tablets, fruit, or granola bars to address potential episodes of hypoglycemia (low blood sugar) during travel.

6. Inform Travel Companions: Inform your travel companions about your diabetes and educate them on the signs and symptoms of hypoglycemia. They can provide support and assistance if needed.

Remember to consult with your healthcare provider before traveling to discuss any specific concerns or recommendations related to your diabetes management during the trip.

Sick-Day Management

Managing diabetes when you're sick requires extra attention and care. Here are some guidelines to help you manage your diabetes during illness:

1. Monitor Blood Sugar: Check your blood sugar levels regularly, as illness can affect your blood sugar levels. Consult with your healthcare provider on the frequency of monitoring and target ranges during illness.

2. Continue Medications: Continue taking your diabetes medications, including insulin or oral medications, as prescribed by your healthcare provider. If you are unable to eat,

discuss alternative medication options with your healthcare team.

3. Stay Hydrated: Drink plenty of fluids, such as water or sugar-free beverages, to prevent dehydration. Aim for regular sips throughout the day.

4. Choose Appropriate Foods: If you have a reduced appetite, try to consume small, frequent meals or snacks that are easy to digest. Opt for foods that won't cause significant blood sugar spikes, such as broth-based soups, plain yogurt, or whole grains.

5. Be Prepared for Ketones: When you're sick, your body may produce ketones, which can be harmful, especially for individuals with type 1 diabetes.

Ketones are detected through a urine or blood test. If you have high ketone levels, seek medical attention promptly.

6. Rest and Prioritize Recovery: Give yourself permission to rest and prioritize your recovery. Allow your body to heal by getting adequate sleep and avoiding overexertion.

It's important to consult with your healthcare provider for personalized advice and sick-day management strategies that are specific to your diabetes type and individual circumstances.

Chapter 9: Preventive Care and Regular Check-ups

Regular medical check-ups and preventive care are essential for effectively managing diabetes and reducing the risk of complications. In this chapter, we will explore the importance of regular check-ups, the significance of eye exams, foot care, dental health, and the role of vaccinations in diabetes management.

Importance of Regular Medical Check-ups

Regular medical check-ups are crucial for individuals with diabetes to monitor their overall health and manage the condition effectively. Here are some reasons why regular check-ups are essential:

1. Monitoring Blood Sugar Levels: Regular check-ups involve monitoring your blood sugar levels through tests such as fasting blood glucose, random blood glucose, and hemoglobin A1c. These tests provide valuable information about your diabetes control and help your healthcare team make necessary adjustments to your treatment plan.

2. Assessing Blood Pressure and Cholesterol Levels: High blood pressure and abnormal cholesterol levels are common among people with diabetes and increase the risk of cardiovascular complications. Regular check-ups allow for the monitoring and management of these conditions to prevent long-term health problems.

3. Detecting Complications Early: Diabetes can lead to various complications that affect different parts of the body, including the eyes, kidneys, nerves, and feet. Regular check-ups help detect early signs of complications, allowing for timely intervention and treatment.

4. Reviewing Medications and Treatment Plan: During check-ups, your healthcare provider will review your current medications, insulin regimen (if applicable), and overall treatment plan. This ensures that your diabetes management is optimized and adjusted as needed.

5. Addressing Lifestyle Factors: Regular check-ups provide an opportunity to

discuss lifestyle factors such as diet, exercise, and stress management. Your healthcare provider can offer guidance and support to help you make positive changes that contribute to better diabetes control.

Eye Exams, Foot Care, and Dental Health

Diabetes can have a significant impact on various aspects of your health, including your eyes, feet, and dental health. Here's why these areas require special attention:

1. Eye Exams: Diabetes increases the risk of eye conditions such as diabetic retinopathy, cataracts, and glaucoma. Regular eye exams help detect any changes in the eyes and enable early treatment to prevent vision loss.

2. Foot Care: Diabetes can cause nerve damage (neuropathy) and poor circulation, increasing the risk of foot problems. Regular foot exams and proper foot care help identify any issues, prevent complications, and promote overall foot health.

3. Dental Health: Diabetes is associated with an increased risk of gum disease (periodontal disease) and other oral health problems. Regular dental check-ups, along with good oral hygiene practices, are crucial for maintaining healthy teeth and gums.

Vaccinations and Diabetes

Vaccinations play an important role in managing diabetes by protecting against infections and preventing related complications. Here are some vaccinations recommended for individuals with diabetes:

1. Influenza (Flu) Vaccine: People with diabetes are at higher risk of developing severe complications from the flu. Annual flu vaccination is recommended to reduce the risk of illness and its impact on diabetes management.

2. Pneumococcal Vaccines: Pneumococcal infections can lead to pneumonia, meningitis, and bloodstream infections. The pneumococcal conjugate vaccine (PCV13) and pneumococcal polysaccharide vaccine (PPSV23) are recommended for individuals with

diabetes to protect against these infections.

3. Hepatitis B Vaccine: Hepatitis B vaccination is important for individuals with diabetes, as they may be at higher risk of contracting the virus through blood glucose monitoring or healthcare procedures. Vaccination helps prevent liver disease and related complications.

4. Other Vaccinations: Depending on individual health status and risk factors, your healthcare provider may recommend additional vaccinations, such as the tetanus-diphtheria-pertussis (Tdap) vaccine, shingles vaccine, or human papillomavirus (HPV) vaccine.

Regular check-ups with your healthcare team will ensure that you are up to date with the recommended vaccinations for your specific situation.

Chapter 10: Diabetes and Special Situations

Living with diabetes presents unique challenges in various life stages and special situations. In this chapter, we will explore diabetes and pregnancy, diabetes in children and adolescents, and aging with diabetes.

Diabetes and Pregnancy

Managing diabetes during pregnancy requires careful monitoring and specialized care. Here are some important considerations:

1. Preconception Planning: If you have diabetes and are planning to conceive, it's essential to work closely with your healthcare team to optimize your blood sugar control before pregnancy. This helps reduce the risk of

complications and promotes a healthy pregnancy.

2. Prenatal Care: During pregnancy, regular prenatal check-ups and close monitoring of blood sugar levels are crucial. Your healthcare provider may adjust your diabetes medications or insulin regimen to maintain optimal control. Additionally, prenatal vitamins and specific dietary recommendations may be prescribed.

3. Gestational Diabetes: Some women develop gestational diabetes during pregnancy, a temporary condition that affects blood sugar levels. Proper management, including a balanced diet, regular physical activity, and blood sugar monitoring, is important

to ensure a healthy pregnancy and minimize potential risks.

4. Potential Risks and Complications: Diabetes during pregnancy can increase the risk of certain complications, such as preeclampsia, preterm birth, and macrosomia (large birth weight). Close monitoring and early intervention help mitigate these risks.

Diabetes in Children and Adolescents

Managing diabetes in children and adolescents requires a collaborative approach involving parents, healthcare providers, and school personnel. Here are key aspects to consider:

1. Type 1 Diabetes in Children: Type 1 diabetes is the most common form of diabetes in children. It requires insulin therapy and careful blood sugar monitoring. Parents play a crucial role in managing their child's diabetes, including administering insulin, monitoring meals, and promoting physical activity.

2. Type 2 Diabetes in Children and Adolescents: The prevalence of type 2 diabetes is increasing among young people, primarily due to lifestyle factors. Treatment often involves a combination of healthy eating, physical activity, oral medications, and, in some cases, insulin therapy.

3. Blood Sugar Monitoring: Regular blood sugar monitoring is essential for children and adolescents with diabetes. Parents and caregivers should work closely with healthcare providers to establish a routine and adjust treatment plans based on blood sugar results.

4. Diabetes Management at School: Communication with school personnel is crucial to ensure a safe and supportive environment for children with diabetes. This may include developing a diabetes management plan, training school staff on diabetes care, and implementing strategies to accommodate blood sugar monitoring, insulin administration, and meal planning.

Aging with Diabetes

As individuals age, diabetes management may become more complex. Here are some important considerations for older adults:

1. Increased Health Risks: Aging with diabetes can increase the risk of other health conditions, such as cardiovascular disease, kidney disease, and cognitive decline. Regular medical check-ups, adherence to medication regimens, and lifestyle modifications are crucial to minimize these risks.

2. Medication Management: Older adults may be taking multiple medications for various health conditions. It's important to work closely with healthcare providers to ensure proper medication management, avoid

potential drug interactions, and monitor for side effects.

3. Nutrition and Physical Activity: Aging adults with diabetes should focus on maintaining a healthy diet that meets their nutritional needs while managing blood sugar levels. Engaging in regular physical activity, as appropriate for their abilities, helps maintain overall health and diabetes control.

4. Preventive Care: Regular preventive care, including vaccinations, eye exams, foot care, and cardiovascular screenings, is vital for older adults with diabetes to prevent complications and maintain their overall well-being.

By understanding and addressing the unique challenges in pregnancy, childhood and adolescence, and aging, individuals with diabetes can navigate these special situations with proper care and support.

Chapter 11: Support and Resources for Diabetes Management

Managing diabetes effectively requires a supportive network and access to valuable resources. In this chapter, we will explore the various support options and resources available to individuals with diabetes.

Diabetes Support Groups and Education Programs

Joining a diabetes support group or participating in diabetes education programs can provide valuable emotional support, practical guidance, and a sense of community. Here are some benefits of these resources:

1. Emotional Support: Diabetes support groups offer a safe space to share experiences, challenges, and triumphs

with others who understand the daily realities of living with diabetes. Connecting with like-minded individuals can provide comfort, encouragement, and a sense of belonging.

2. Knowledge and Education: Diabetes education programs provide comprehensive information about diabetes management, including self-care techniques, medication management, blood sugar monitoring, and lifestyle modifications. These programs empower individuals with the knowledge and skills to effectively manage their diabetes.

3. Practical Tips and Strategies: Support groups and education programs often

include discussions, workshops, and guest speakers who provide practical tips and strategies for managing diabetes in real-life situations. Participants can learn from others' experiences and gain insights into successful diabetes management approaches.

Online Resources and Mobile Applications

The digital age has brought forth a wealth of online resources and mobile applications that can support diabetes management. Here are some ways these resources can be beneficial:

1. Information and Education: Reliable websites, blogs, and online forums offer a wealth of information about

diabetes, treatment options, self-care tips, and the latest research. These resources can help individuals stay informed and up to date with advancements in diabetes management.

2. Blood Sugar Tracking: Numerous mobile applications are available to track blood sugar levels, record medications and meals, and generate reports for analysis. These apps make it convenient to monitor diabetes-related data and share it with healthcare providers for better treatment decisions.

3. Nutrition and Meal Planning: Online platforms and mobile apps offer access to nutritional information,

recipe ideas, meal planning tools, and personalized meal tracking features. These resources help individuals make informed food choices, manage their carbohydrate intake, and maintain a balanced diet.

4. Community and Support: Online diabetes communities and social media groups provide a platform to connect with individuals worldwide who are living with diabetes. These communities offer support, share experiences, and provide a sense of belonging and understanding.

Financial Assistance and Insurance Coverage

Managing diabetes can be financially challenging, but there are resources available to help individuals access the necessary healthcare and diabetes supplies. Here are some options to consider:

1. Health Insurance Coverage: Understanding your health insurance coverage and benefits is crucial. Review your policy to determine coverage for diabetes-related medications, supplies, and medical services. Speak with your insurance provider or employer's human resources department for clarification and assistance.

2. Prescription Assistance Programs: Pharmaceutical companies and nonprofit organizations offer prescription assistance programs that provide discounts or free medications

to eligible individuals who meet specific criteria. These programs can help reduce the financial burden of diabetes medications.

3. Financial Assistance Programs: There are financial assistance programs available that provide support for diabetes-related expenses, including supplies, devices, and educational resources. Research and inquire about local and national programs that may offer financial aid to individuals with diabetes.

4. Patient Assistance Programs: Some pharmaceutical companies offer patient assistance programs that provide medications at reduced or no cost for eligible individuals who meet

specific income criteria. These programs help ensure access to essential diabetes medications.

By utilizing the support groups, education programs, online resources, and financial assistance options available, individuals with diabetes can enhance their knowledge, find emotional support, and overcome financial barriers to effective diabetes management.

Conclusion

Empowering Yourself for Optimal Diabetes Management

Managing diabetes is a lifelong journey that requires dedication, knowledge, and a proactive approach. By understanding the essential principles of diabetes management and adopting a comprehensive approach to your health and well-being, you can empower yourself to live a fulfilling life while effectively managing your diabetes.

Throughout this comprehensive handbook, we have explored various aspects of diabetes management, from understanding the condition and its causes to practical strategies for maintaining optimal health and wellness. We have covered topics such as:

- The fundamentals of diabetes, including types, symptoms, and risk factors.

- The importance of regular medical check-ups and preventive care.

- Strategies for managing blood sugar levels through nutrition, physical activity, and medication.

- The benefits of exercise, creating an exercise plan, and incorporating physical activity into daily life.

- Medications and insulin therapy options for diabetes management.

- Techniques for monitoring blood sugar levels and interpreting readings.

- Coping with stress, emotional challenges, and special situations such as travel and sick-day management.

- Diabetes management during pregnancy, in children and adolescents, and as you age.

- The significance of support groups, education programs, online resources, and financial assistance in diabetes management.

By adopting the strategies, tools, and resources outlined in this handbook, you can take charge of your diabetes management journey and strive for optimal health and wellness. Remember that diabetes management is highly individualized, and it's essential to work closely with your healthcare team to develop a personalized plan that meets your unique needs.

Additional Resources: To further support your diabetes management journey, consider exploring the following resources:

1. Diabetes Associations and Organizations: National and local diabetes associations and organizations offer a wealth of information, resources, and support

for individuals with diabetes. Examples include the American Diabetes Association (ADA), Diabetes UK, and the International Diabetes Federation (IDF).

2. Books and Publications: Numerous books and publications are available that delve deeper into specific aspects of diabetes management. Look for reputable titles written by healthcare professionals, diabetes educators, and individuals with personal experience in managing diabetes.

3. Online Communities and Forums: Engaging with online communities and forums dedicated to diabetes can provide a platform for sharing experiences, asking questions, and

gaining support from individuals who understand the challenges of living with diabetes.

4. Mobile Applications: Explore diabetes-specific mobile applications that can help you track blood sugar levels, manage medications, monitor meals, and provide educational resources on the go.

5. Diabetes Education Programs: Consider enrolling in diabetes education programs offered by healthcare providers, hospitals, and community centers. These programs provide valuable information, practical skills, and support from healthcare professionals and educators.

Remember, diabetes management is a continuous learning process. Stay proactive, stay informed, and take the necessary steps to prioritize your health and well-being. With proper self-care, a supportive network, and access to valuable resources, you can lead a fulfilling life while effectively managing your diabetes.

At NeoLife, we are committed to providing innovative solutions for optimal health and well-being. As you embark on your journey to manage diabetes and achieve optimal wellness, we would like to introduce you to our range of high-quality nutritional products designed to support your overall health goals.

Our scientifically advanced supplements, including our popular **NeoLifeShake**, provide essential nutrients, vitamins, and minerals that can complement your diabetes management plan. With a focus on quality and efficacy, our products undergo rigorous testing and adhere to the highest industry standards.

We believe that nutrition plays a vital role in maintaining stable blood sugar levels, supporting cardiovascular health, and promoting overall vitality. That's why our products are formulated with the finest ingredients, carefully selected for their nutritional benefits.

To explore our full range of products and learn how they can support your journey toward optimal health and diabetes management, visit our website at https://shopneolife.com/olanrewajuganiyu. As a valued reader of "The Essential Guide to Managing Diabetes," we would like to see you live a fulfilled and healthy life which is why we are bringing to you a full pack support and information.

Remember, managing diabetes is a holistic endeavor, and proper nutrition is a cornerstone of that journey. NeoLife is here to support you every step of the way. Together, let's unlock the power of nutrition and achieve a life of vibrant health and well-being.